OH, BABY!

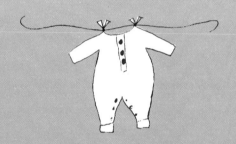

Project editor: S A N D R A   G I L B E R T
Production: K I M   T Y N E R

Published in 2001 by
Stewart, Tabori & Chang
115 West 18th Street
New York, NY 10011
www.abramsbooks.com

ISBN: 1-58479-038-5

Printed in China

10 9 8 7 6 5 4 3

Designed by N I N A   B A R N E T T

Stewart, Tabori & Chang is a subsidiary of
LA MARTINIÈRE
GROUPE

OH, BABY!

A JOURNAL

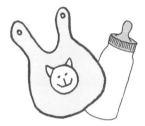

by **HÉLÈNE TRAGOS STELIAN**

illustrated by **THERESA CASE**

Stewart, Tabori & Chang
New York

TO _____

FROM _____

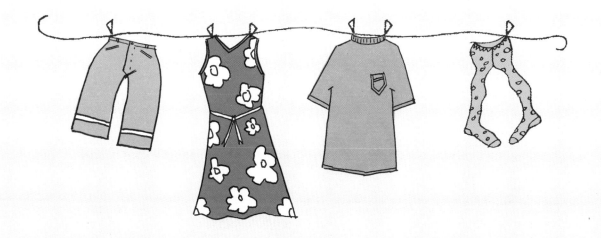

YOUR FAMILY

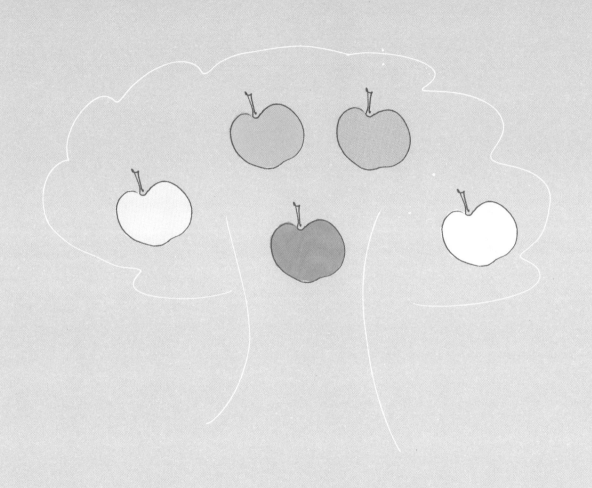

YOUR family history

_____

_____

_____

_____

_____

_____

_____

_____

_____

_____

MOMMY'S family tree

Mommy _____

Birthplace _____ Date _____

Your grandmother _____ Your grandfather _____

Birthplace _____ Birthplace _____

Date _____ Date _____

Your aunts _____

Your uncles _____

Your cousins _____

_____

DADDY'S family tree

Daddy _____

Birthplace _____ Date _____

Your grandmother _____ Your grandfather _____

Birthplace _____ Birthplace _____

Date _____ Date _____

Your aunts _____

Your uncles _____

Your cousins _____

_____

MOMMY and DADDY

Meeting EACH OTHER

_____

_____

_____

_____

Our personalities, careers, and interests

_____

_____

_____

_____

PHOTO

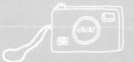

click!

HERE

_____

DATE

AWAITING YOU

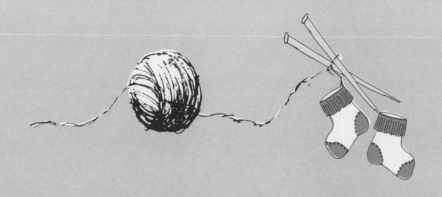

FINDING OUT about you

HEARING and SHARING the news

_____

_____

_____

_____

_____

_____

_____

_____

_____

_____

EXPECTING you

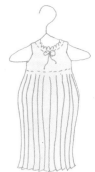

Mommy's FEELINGS and CRAVINGS

_____

_____

_____

_____

Daddy's TURN

_____

_____

_____

_____

MOMMY'S BELLY PHOTO or

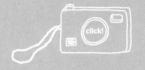

ULTRASOUND HERE

_____

DATE and AGE

FEELING you

Your HEARTBEAT, your KICKS

_____

_____

_____

_____

A BOY or a GIRL

_____

_____

_____

_____

preparations

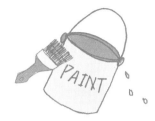

SHOPPING for you, DECORATING your nursery

_____

_____

_____

_____

CHILDBIRTH and PARENTING classes

_____

_____

_____

_____

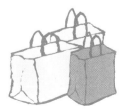

the BABY SHOWER

In Honor of _____

When _____

Where _____

Given by _____

Guests _____

_____

Favorite moments _____

_____

Memorable gifts _____

_____

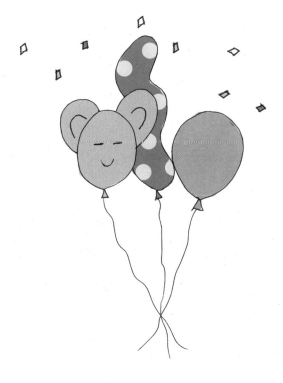

WELCOME

your ARRIVAL

Baby's Name _____

Date _____ Time _____

Weight _____ Length _____

Where you were born

_____

_____

_____

Doctor, midwife, others attending

_____

_____

_____

PHOTO

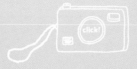

HERE

_____

DATE

your BIRTH STORY

As told by MOMMY

_____

_____

_____

_____

_____

_____

_____

_____

_____

_____

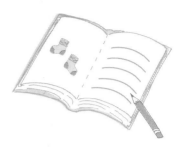

DADDY'S turn

_____

_____

_____

_____

_____

_____

_____

_____

_____

_____

FIRST FAMILY

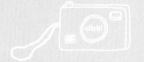

PHOTO HERE

_____

DATE

first IMPRESSIONS

The color of your EYES, the feel of your SKIN

_____

_____

_____

You LOOK like

_____

_____

_____

Our THOUGHTS and FEELINGS

_____

_____

_____

your N A M E

SIGNIFICANCE

NICKNAMES

RUNNERS-UP

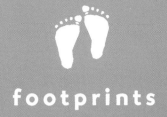

footprints

_____

DATE

mementos

HOSPITAL BRACELET and OTHER KEEPSAKES

the **YEAR** you were **BORN**

Major NEWS STORIES

_____

_____

_____

_____

Other EVENTS

_____

_____

_____

_____

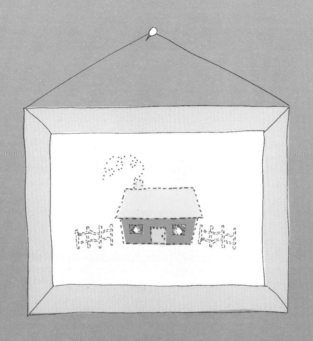

HOME SWEET HOME

your first home

PHOTO

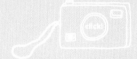

HERE

_____

DATE

WELCOME home

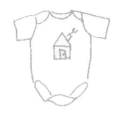

Bringing you HOME

Your first ADDRESS

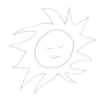

your first **WEEK**

Early DAYS and NIGHTS

_____

_____

_____

_____

_____

_____

_____

_____

_____

your first VISITORS

Who they were, what they said

CELEBRATING you

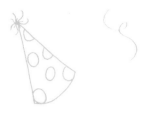

Gatherings, parties, and ceremonies

PHOTO

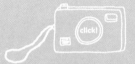

HERE

_____

DATE and AGE

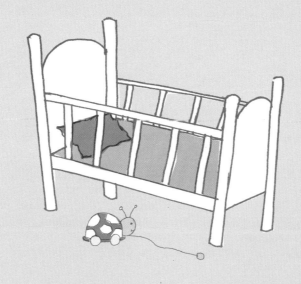

SETTLING IN

PHOTO

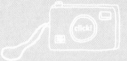

HERE

_____

DATE and AGE

LULLABY

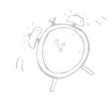

Your SLEEP schedule

_____

_____

_____

Sleeping through the NIGHT

_____

_____

_____

Bedtime RITUALS

_____

_____

_____

MEALTIME

What you ATE, when, and how

_____

_____

_____

_____

_____

_____

_____

_____

_____

_____

PHOTO

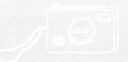

HERE

_____

DATE and AGE

PHOTO

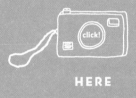

HERE

DATE and AGE

getting **MESSY**

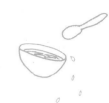

Your first SOLID FOODS and FINGER FOODS

_____

_____

_____

Holding your own BOTTLE, your own SPOON

_____

_____

_____

First meal in a RESTAURANT

_____

_____

_____

TUB time

Your first BATH

_____

_____

_____

_____

Bath-time RITUALS

_____

_____

_____

_____

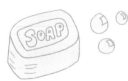

PHOTO

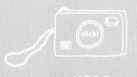

HERE

_____

DATE and AGE

your first haircut

LOCK OF HAIR

DATE and AGE

favorite OUTFITS

From SLEEPERS to overalls, BOOTIES to shoes

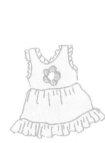

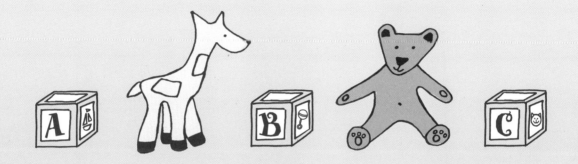

PLAYTIME

favorites

Toys and stuffed animals _____

Lullabies and songs _____

Games and rhymes _____

Books and videos _____

Security objects such as blankies and pacifiers _____

Classes and playgroups _____

Pets and little friends _____

PHOTO

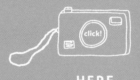

HERE

_____

DATE and AGE

PHOTO

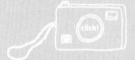

HERE

DATE and AGE

time with MOMMY

Favorite RITUALS and fun GAMES

_____

_____

_____

_____

Only MOMMY can . . .

_____

_____

_____

_____

time with DADDY

Favorite RITUALS and fun GAMES

_____

_____

_____

_____

Only DADDY can . . .

_____

_____

_____

_____

PHOTO

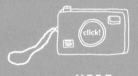

HERE

_____

DATE and AGE

doodles and scribbles

PASTE IN HERE

_____

DATE and AGE

outings

First trips to the park, zoo, and pool

_____

_____

_____

First experiences with rain and snow

_____

_____

_____

First vacation

_____

_____

_____

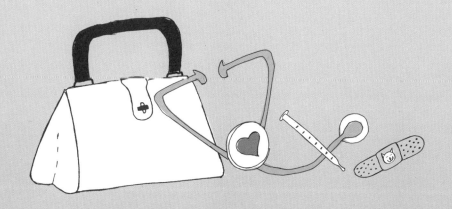

HEALTHY BABY

visiting the DOCTOR

IMMUNIZATIONS AND TESTS

Type	Date	Notes

ILLNESSES AND MISHAPS

Type	Date	Notes

sooo BIG

	WEIGHT	LENGTH
Birth		
2 weeks		
1 month		
2 months		
3 months		
4 months		
5 months		
6 months		
7 months		
8 months		
9 months		
10 months		
11 months		
1 year		

your first **TOOTH**

Your first tooth appeared

_____

_____

_____

We knew you were teething when

_____

_____

_____

Reactions and soothers

_____

_____

_____

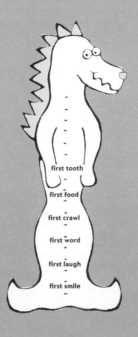

first tooth

first food

first crawl

first word

first laugh

first smile

MILESTONES

FIRSTS

	AGE	NOTES

You lifted your head up _____

You rolled over _____

You sat unassisted _____

You crawled _____

You pulled up to stand _____

You stood unassisted _____

You cruised _____

You took your first steps _____

	AGE	NOTES

You followed an object with your eyes _____

You found your fingers and toes _____

You grasped a rattle _____

You pointed _____

You waved bye-bye _____

You clapped your hands _____

You rolled a ball _____

You grasped with your thumb and finger _____

FUNNY baby

Your first smile and laugh

_____

_____

_____

What makes you smile and laugh

_____

_____

_____

Funny things you do

_____

_____

_____

PHOTO

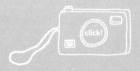

HERE

_____

DATE and AGE

CHATTY baby

Cooing, BABBLING, first words

_____

_____

_____

_____

_____

_____

_____

_____

_____

_____

NAUGHTY baby

Playful PLOTS, favorite TRICKS

_____

_____

_____

_____

_____

_____

_____

_____

_____

_____

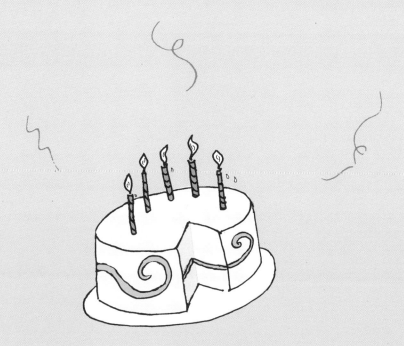

SPECIAL DAYS

holidays

Celebrations with you

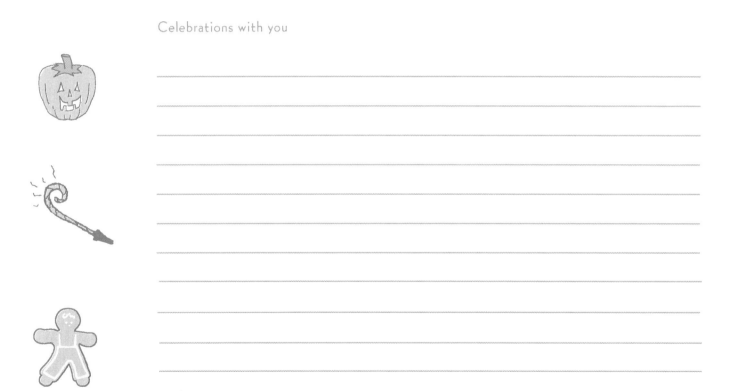

PHOTO

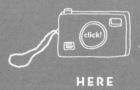

HERE

_____

DATE and AGE

PHOTO

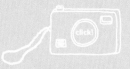

HERE

_____

DATE and AGE

first **BIRTHDAY**

When and where

_____

_____

_____

Guests

_____

_____

_____

Memorable moments and gifts

_____

_____

_____

highlights of

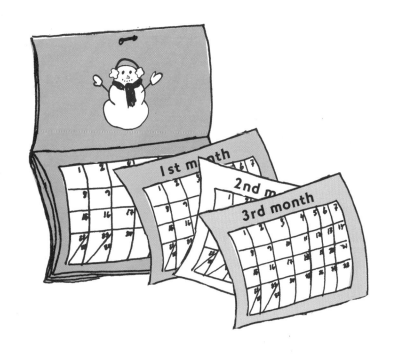

YOUR FIRST YEAR

OH, BABY grow!

month _____

_____

_____

2 months _____

_____

_____

3 months _____

_____

_____

more adventures and discoveries

4 months _____
_____
_____

5 months _____
_____
_____

6 months _____
_____
_____

7

months _____

_____

_____

8

months _____

_____

_____

9

months _____

_____

_____

10
months _____

_____

_____

11
months _____

_____

_____

12
months _____

_____

_____

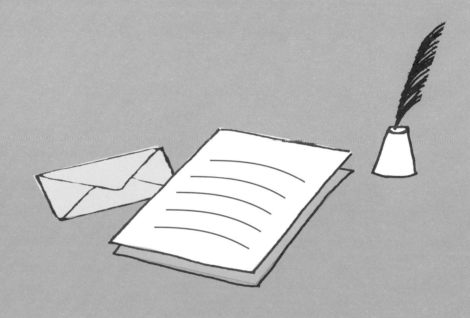

FAN MAIL

FAN mail

Letter from MOMMY

_____

_____

_____

_____

_____

_____

_____

_____

_____

_____

DADDY'S turn

FAN mail

Letter from a relative, friend, or sitter

_____

_____

_____

_____

_____

_____

_____

_____

_____

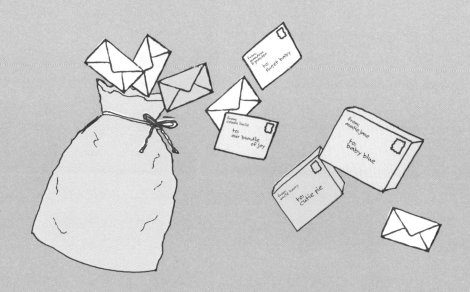

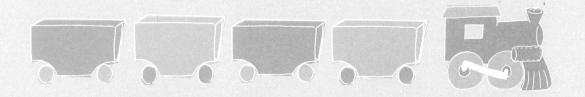